Blood Type O Diet Recipes for Beginners

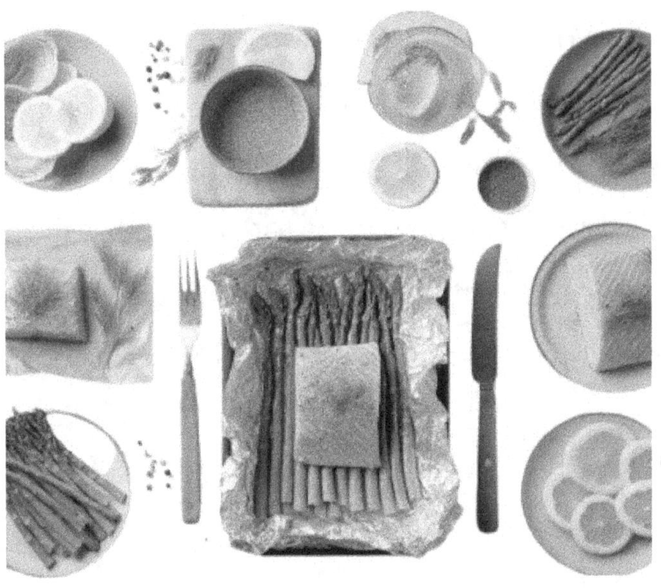

A Personalized Cookbook with Easy and Healthy Recipes for Your Blood Type

LANITA CRUZ

Copyright © 2023 by Lanita Cruz

TABLE OF CONTENTS

DISCLAIMER

The recipes and information provided in "Blood Type O Diet Recipes for Beginners" are intended for informational and educational purposes only and not as a substitute for professional medical advice, diagnosis, or treatment. While these recipes align with the Blood Type O diet principles, individual dietary needs may vary.

It is advisable to consult with a healthcare professional or a registered dietitian before making significant changes to your diet, especially if you have health conditions or concerns. The author and publisher are not responsible for any adverse effects or consequences resulting from the use or misuse of the information in this cookbook. Always use caution and make informed choices based on your unique health circumstances.

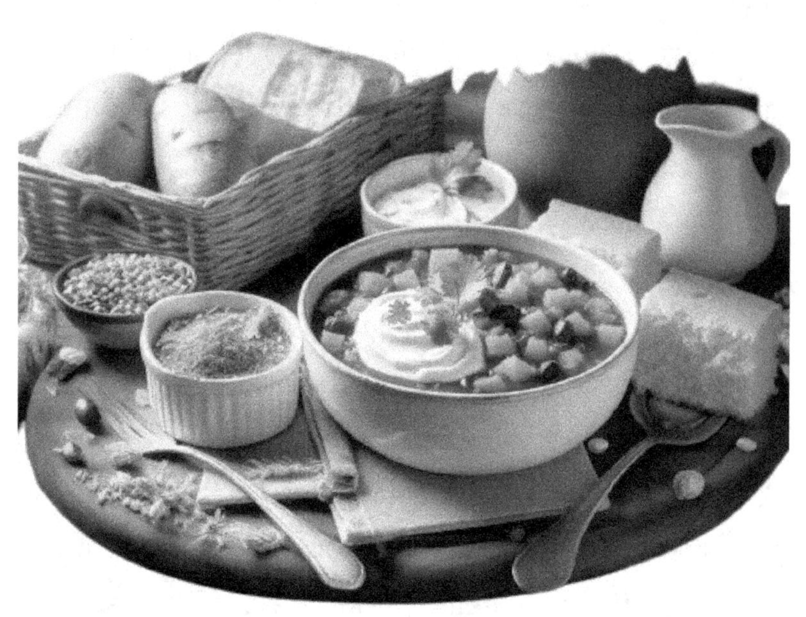

Introduction

This is "Blood Type O Diet Recipes for Beginners," a cookbook that will help you discover the best foods for your blood type and how to prepare them in delicious and easy ways.

Ever wondered why some diets work wonders for some but not for others? The answer you seek may lie in your blood type. The Blood Type O Diet is a personalized approach to nutrition, acknowledging that individuals with Blood Type O may thrive on specific foods while others may hinder their well-being.

If you have blood type O, you may have heard that following a diet that suits your blood type can improve your health, boost your energy, and prevent diseases. As we delve into this dietary philosophy, you'll discover the science behind it and how tailoring your meals to your blood type can be a game-changer.

The journey to optimal health isn't just about the food on your plate; it's about understanding how your body responds to it. In this cookbook, I explore the benefits of the Blood Type O Diet, from improved digestion to enhanced metabolism.

By embracing the right foods and avoiding the ones that may not serve you well, you're not just nourishing your body; you're embracing a lifestyle that aligns with your unique genetic makeup.

In this cookbook, you will find everything you need to know about the blood type O diet, including the benefits, the tips and advice, the grocery shopping list, the beneficial and harmful foods, and of course, the recipes.

You will learn how to make tasty and nutritious meals for breakfast, lunch, and dinner, as well as desserts, snacks, and beverages that are suitable for your blood type. You will also get a 30-day meal plan that will help you plan your meals and stick to your diet.

Whether you are new to the blood type O diet or you have been following it for a while, this cookbook will provide you with a variety of recipes that will satisfy your taste buds and your health goals.

So, are you ready to start your journey to a healthier and happier life with the blood type O diet? Let's begin!

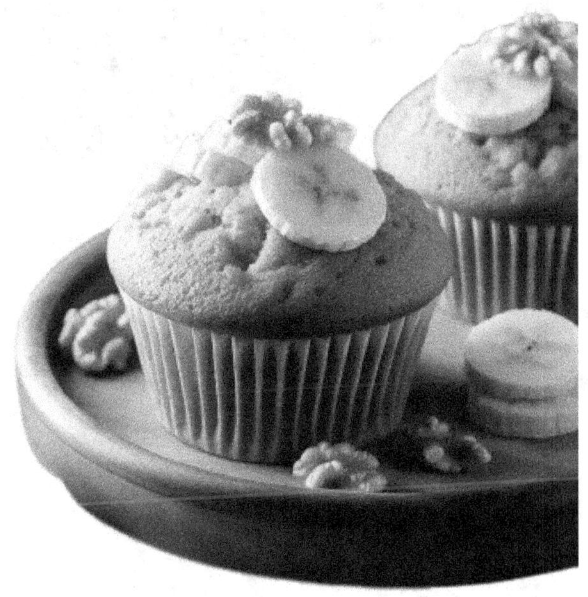

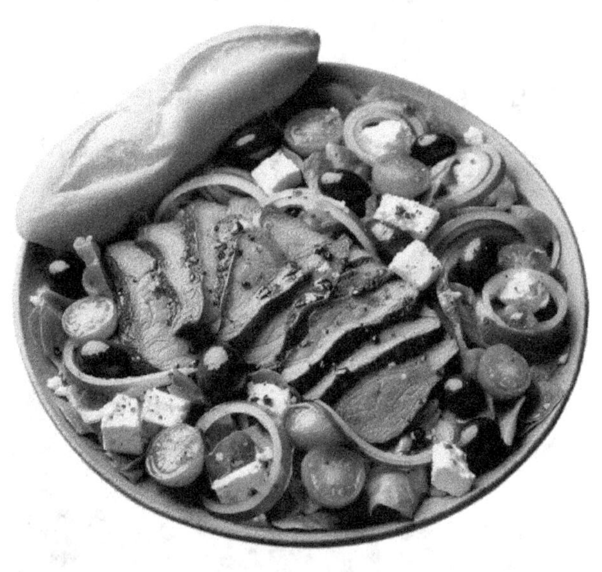

CHAPTER 1

Benefits of the Blood Type O Diet

Embarking on the Blood Type O Diet isn't just a journey through delicious recipes; it's a commitment to unlocking a wealth of health benefits uniquely tailored to individuals with Blood Type O. Here are some of the benefits of aligning your diet with your blood type:

1. *Enhanced Metabolism:* Your blood type influences how efficiently your body processes and metabolizes food. For Blood Type O individuals, embracing the recommended foods can kickstart and optimize metabolism, leading to increased energy levels and effective weight management.

2. *Improved Digestion:* The key to overall well-being often lies in the digestive system. By aligning your diet with your blood type, you support a digestive environment that promotes nutrient absorption, reduces bloating, and minimizes digestive discomfort.

3. *Immune System Support:* The foods you consume play a crucial role in supporting your immune system. With the Blood Type O Diet, you'll discover a selection of foods that may enhance your body's ability to fend off illnesses, keeping you feeling strong and resilient.

4. *Weight Management:* Shedding excess weight and maintaining a healthy body composition is a common goal. By understanding the foods that complement your blood type, you can create a sustainable and effective approach to weight management that goes beyond temporary fixes.

5. *Increased Energy Levels:* Imagine waking up with a renewed sense of energy, ready to conquer the day. The Blood Type O Diet aims to provide the necessary nutrients to fuel your body, helping you maintain consistent energy levels throughout the day.

6. *Balanced Hormones:* Hormones play a crucial role in various bodily functions, from mood regulation to metabolism. By embracing the right foods, you can contribute to hormonal balance, promoting emotional well-being and overall harmony within your body.

7. *Optimal Cardiovascular Health:* Heart health is paramount, and the Blood Type O Diet emphasizes foods that may positively impact cardiovascular health. From supporting healthy blood circulation to managing cholesterol levels, these dietary choices contribute to a heart-healthy lifestyle.

Tips and Advice on How to Follow the Blood Type O Diet

1. *Know Your Blood Type:* Before you embark on this culinary adventure, it's essential to know your blood type. Understanding whether you are Blood Type O lays the foundation for tailoring your diet to your unique biological makeup.

2. *Familiarize Yourself with Beneficial and Avoid Foods:* One of the cornerstones of the Blood Type O Diet is recognizing which foods are beneficial, neutral, or best avoided. Familiarize yourself with the comprehensive list provided in this cookbook to make informed choices.

3. Embrace Variety in Your Diet: While certain foods are emphasized for Blood Type O, variety is key to a well-rounded and nutritious diet. Explore a diverse range of vegetables, proteins, and grains to ensure you get a spectrum of nutrients.

4. Plan Your Meals Ahead: Planning is a powerful tool on your journey to success. Develop a weekly meal plan, incorporating a balance of breakfasts, lunches, dinners, and snacks. This not only helps with grocery shopping but also ensures you have Blood Type O-friendly options readily available.

5. Master the Art of Grocery Shopping: Armed with your knowledge of beneficial foods, navigate the grocery store with confidence. Stick to the perimeter, where fresh produce and lean proteins are usually located, and refer to your Blood Type O Grocery Shopping List for guidance.

6. *Prepare Flavorful Blood Type O-Friendly Recipes:* The heart of the Blood Type O Diet lies in the kitchen. Experiment with the diverse and delicious recipes provided in this cookbook. From breakfast to dinner, each dish is crafted to satisfy your palate while adhering to the principles of the Blood Type O Diet.

7. *Listen to Your Body:* Pay attention to how your body responds to different foods. The Blood Type O Diet is a guide, but your body is the ultimate navigator. If you notice positive changes or sensitivities, adjust your diet accordingly.

8. *Stay Hydrated:* Adequate hydration is essential for overall health. While water is universally beneficial, consider incorporating beverages that align with the Blood Type O recommendations, such as herbal teas or fruit-infused water.

9. *Find Support and Stay Motivated:* Share your journey with friends or family members who may also be exploring the Blood Type O Diet. Having a support system can provide encouragement and motivation on your path to wellness.

10. Celebrate Your Progress: Every step forward is a victory. Celebrate your successes, whether they are small dietary changes, increased energy levels, or improved well-being. Acknowledge and appreciate the positive impact you're making on your health.

Grocery Shopping List for Blood Type O

Proteins:

1. Lean cuts of beef
2. Lamb
3. Turkey
4. Chicken
5. Fish (especially cold-water varieties like salmon and mackerel)
6. Eggs

Vegetables: 7. Kale

8. Spinach
9. Broccoli
10. Sweet potatoes
11. Onions

12. Garlic

13. Bell peppers

Fruits: 14. Berries (blueberries, strawberries, raspberries)

15. Cherries

16. Plums

17. Figs

18. Prunes

Grains: 19. Quinoa

20. Brown rice

21. Millet

Legumes: 22. Lentils

23. Black-eyed peas

Dairy and Alternatives: 24. Goat cheese

25. Feta cheese

26. Almond milk

Nuts and Seeds: 27. Walnuts

28. Pumpkin seeds

29. Flaxseeds

Oils: 30. Olive oil

31. Flaxseed oil

Herbs and Spices: 32. Turmeric

33. Ginger

34. Parsley

35. Rosemary

36. Thyme

Condiments: 37. Tamari sauce (gluten-free soy sauce)

38. Mustard

Beverages: 39. Green tea

40. Herbal teas

Sweeteners: 41. Agave nectar

42. Maple syrup

Additional Items: 43. Sea salt

44. Black pepper

45. Vinegar (especially apple cider vinegar)

This comprehensive Grocery Shopping List is designed to simplify your shopping experience, ensuring that you have the essentials to create delicious and Blood Type O-friendly meals. As you stroll through the aisles, refer to this list to make informed choices, and let the vibrant colors of fresh produce guide you toward optimal health.

Beneficial Foods for Blood Type O

From nutrient-rich proteins to vibrant vegetables, let's explore the key players that make this culinary journey both delicious and health-enhancing.

1. Lean Proteins:

- Beef: Go for lean cuts like sirloin or tenderloin.
- Lamb: A flavorful and nutrient-rich protein source.

- Turkey: A versatile and lean poultry option.
- Chicken: Choose skinless, lean cuts for a protein boost.
- Fish: Particularly cold-water varieties like salmon and mackerel, rich in omega-3 fatty acids.
- Eggs: A protein-packed option with essential vitamins.

2. Nutrient-Dense Vegetables:

- Kale: Packed with vitamins, minerals, and antioxidants.
- Spinach: A versatile leafy green with a wealth of nutrients.
- Broccoli: Rich in fiber, vitamins, and immune-boosting properties.
- Sweet Potatoes: A complex carbohydrate with a sweet and savory flair.
- Onions: Add flavor and potential anti-inflammatory benefits.
- Garlic: This is popular for its heart-healthy and immune-boosting properties.

- Bell Peppers: Colorful and rich in vitamins.

3. Berries and Cherries:

- Blueberries, Strawberries, Raspberries: Bursting with antioxidants and vitamins.
- Cherries: Known for their anti-inflammatory properties.

4. Figs and Plums:

- Figs: A sweet and nutritious addition, high in fiber.
- Plums: Rich in antioxidants and a good source of vitamins.

5. Quinoa and Brown Rice:

- Quinoa: A complete protein with a nutty flavor.
- Brown Rice: A whole grain providing essential nutrients.

6. Lentils and Black-Eyed Peas:

- Lentils: High in protein, fiber, and various vitamins.
- Black-Eyed Peas: A good source of folate, potassium, and iron.

7. Goat and Feta Cheese:

- Goat Cheese: A flavorful and easily digestible dairy option.
- Feta Cheese: Adds a tangy kick to salads and dishes.

8. Healthy Fats:

- Walnuts: Packed with omega-3 fatty acids and antioxidants.
- Flaxseeds: A rich source of omega-3s and fiber.
- Olive Oil: A heart-healthy oil with anti-inflammatory properties.

9. Herbs and Spices:

- Turmeric: Known for its anti-inflammatory properties.

- Ginger: Adds warmth and potential digestive benefits.
- Parsley, Rosemary, Thyme: Flavorful herbs with potential health benefits.

10. Beverages:

- Green Tea: Rich in antioxidants and associated with various health benefits.
- Herbal Teas: Choose caffeine-free varieties for a soothing option.

Foods to Avoid

While the Blood Type O Diet emphasizes beneficial foods that align with your unique physiology, it's equally important to be aware of items that may not harmonize well with your blood type.

1. Dairy Products:

- Cow's Milk: Contains lectins that may not be well-tolerated.
- American Cheese: Often highly processed and may contain additives.

2. Grains:

- Wheat: Contains lectins and gluten, which may be challenging for Blood Type O.
- Corn: Best avoided due to its lectin content.
- Barley: Contains gluten and may be less compatible.

3. Legumes:

- Kidney Beans: High in lectins that may interfere with digestion.
- Navy Beans: Another lectin-rich legume best avoided.
- Lentils (in excess): While lentils are beneficial in moderation, excessive consumption may pose challenges.

4. Certain Fruits:

- Oranges: The lectin content in oranges may not align well with Blood Type O.

- Strawberries (in excess): While berries are generally beneficial, excessive strawberries may be best limited.

5. Processed Meats:

- Bacon: Often processed and high in additives.
- Ham: Processed and may contain additives that are less compatible.

6. High-Fat Dairy:

- Whole Milk: High in saturated fats.
- Ice Cream: Contains both dairy and added sugars.

7. Processed and Refined Foods:

- Highly Processed Snacks: Often contain additives and preservatives.
- Packaged Convenience Foods: May contain ingredients less suitable for Blood Type O.

8. Certain Vegetables:

- Brussels Sprouts: May interfere with thyroid function for some Blood Type O individuals.
- Cauliflower: Best consumed in moderation due to its impact on thyroid function.

9. Shellfish:

- Crab and Lobster: May not be the ideal protein source for Blood Type O.

10. Certain Beverages:

- Soda: High in sugars and additives.
- Black Tea (in excess): While moderate amounts may be acceptable, excessive consumption may pose challenges.

Remember, the key to success with the Blood Type O Diet is balance and awareness of how your body responds to different foods. By avoiding items that may not align with your blood type, you create a foundation for optimal health and well-being.

CHAPTER 2

Breakfast Recipes for Blood Type O

Beef and Vegetable Stir-Fry with Buckwheat Noodles

Preparation Time: 20 minutes

Serves: 2

Ingredients:

- 200g lean beef, thinly sliced
- 150g buckwheat noodles
- 1 cup broccoli florets
- 1 bell pepper, thinly sliced
- 1 carrot, julienned
- 2 tablespoons tamari sauce
- 1 tablespoon sesame oil
- 1 tablespoon olive oil
- 2 cloves garlic, minced
- 1 teaspoon ginger, grated
- Sesame seeds for garnish (optional)
- Green onions for garnish (optional)

Nutritional Information: Calories: 400kcal | Protein: 25g | Carbohydrates: 45g | Fat: 15g | Fiber: 8g

Instructions:

1. Cook buckwheat noodles according to package instructions, then drain and set aside.
2. Heat olive oil in a wok or large skillet over medium-high heat.
3. Add thinly sliced beef and stir-fry until browned. Remove it from the wok and keep it aside.
4. In the same wok, add sesame oil and sauté garlic and ginger until fragrant.
5. Add broccoli, bell pepper, and julienned carrot. Stir-fry for 3-4 minutes until vegetables are crisp-tender.
6. Return the cooked beef to the wok, add tamari sauce, and toss to combine.
7. Add the cooked buckwheat noodles, tossing until well-coated and heated through.
8. Add sesame seeds and green onions as garnish if you like.
9. Serve immediately.

Serving Suggestions:

- If you like, top it off with additional fresh herbs like cilantro or basil.
- For added heat, sprinkle red pepper flakes before serving.
- Pair with a side of kimchi for a probiotic boost.

Buckwheat Pancakes with Berry Compote

Preparation Time: 15 minutes

Serves: 2

Ingredients:

- 1 cup buckwheat flour
- 1 teaspoon baking powder
- 1/2 teaspoon cinnamon
- 1 cup almond milk
- 1 large egg
- 2 tablespoons maple syrup
- 1 teaspoon vanilla extract
- Coconut oil for cooking

Nutritional Information: Calories: 350kcal | Protein: 10g | Carbohydrates: 60g | Fat: 8g | Fiber: 8g

Instructions:

1. In a mixing bowl, combine buckwheat flour, baking powder, and cinnamon.
2. In a separate bowl, whisk together almond milk, egg, maple syrup, and vanilla extract.
3. Combine the wet ingredients with the dry ingredients and stir until just mixed.
4. Heat a skillet or griddle over medium heat and lightly coat with coconut oil.
5. Pour 1/4 cup of batter for each pancake onto the hot surface.
6. Continue cooking until you see bubbles on the surface, then flip and cook the opposite side until it achieves a golden brown color.
7. Repeat until all batter is used.
8. Serve pancakes warm with the Berry Compote.

Berry Compote:

- 1 cup mixed berries (blueberries, strawberries, raspberries)

- 1 tablespoon chia seeds

- 1 tablespoon maple syrup

Nutritional Information (Berry Compote): Calories: 60kcal | Protein: 1g | Carbohydrates: 15g | Fat: 1g | Fiber: 3g

Instructions (Berry Compote):

1. In a saucepan, combine mixed berries, chia seeds, and maple syrup.
2. Simmer over low heat, stirring occasionally, until the berries break down and the mixture thickens (about 8-10 minutes).
3. Remove from heat and let it cool slightly before serving over the Buckwheat Pancakes.

Serving Suggestions:

- Top pancakes with a dollop of Greek yogurt for added protein.
- Sprinkle chopped nuts like almonds or walnuts for a crunchy texture.
- Drizzle extra maple syrup or honey for those with a sweeter tooth.

Broccoli and Feta Frittata

Preparation Time: 25 minutes

Serves: 4

Ingredients:

- 6 large eggs
- 1 cup broccoli florets, steamed
- 1/2 cup crumbled feta cheese
- 1/4 cup diced red onion
- 1 tablespoon olive oil
- Salt and pepper to taste
- Fresh parsley for garnish (optional)

Nutritional Information: Calories: 220kcal | Protein: 15g | Carbohydrates: 5g | Fat: 16g | Fiber: 2g

Instructions:

1. Preheat the oven to 375°F (190°C).
2. In a bowl, whisk together eggs, salt, and pepper until well combined.
3. Warm olive oil in an oven-safe skillet set to medium heat.
4. Add diced red onion and sauté until translucent.

5. Add steamed broccoli florets to the skillet, spreading them evenly.

6. Pour the whisked eggs over the broccoli and onion mixture.

7. Sprinkle crumbled feta evenly across the frittata.

8. Cook on the stovetop for 2-3 minutes, allowing the edges to set.

9. Transfer the skillet to the preheated oven and bake for 15-18 minutes or until the frittata is set and slightly golden.

10. Remove from the oven and let it cool briefly before slicing.

11. Garnish with fresh parsley if desired.

Serving Suggestions:

- Serve with a side of mixed greens for a light lunch.
- Pair with a slice of whole-grain toast for added fiber.
- Drizzle with hot sauce for a spicy kick.

Almond Flour Pancakes

Preparation Time: 15 minutes

Serves: 2

Ingredients:

- 1 cup almond flour
- 1/2 teaspoon baking powder
- 2 large eggs
- 1/4 cup almond milk
- 1 tablespoon coconut oil, melted
- 1 tablespoon maple syrup (plus extra for serving)
- 1 teaspoon vanilla extract
- Pinch of salt

Nutritional Information: Calories: 380kcal | Protein: 14g | Carbohydrates: 14g | Fat: 32g | Fiber: 6g

Instructions:

1. In a bowl, whisk together almond flour, baking powder, and a pinch of salt.
2. In a separate bowl, beat the eggs and add almond milk, melted coconut oil, maple syrup, and vanilla extract. Mix well.

3. Combine the wet and dry ingredients, stirring until a smooth batter forms.

4. Warm a skillet or griddle on medium heat and lightly coat with coconut oil.

5. Pour 1/4 cup of batter for each pancake onto the hot surface.

6. Continue cooking until you see bubbles on the surface, then flip and cook the opposite side until it achieves a golden brown color.

7. Repeat until all batter is used.

8. Serve the pancakes while warm, topped with a drizzle of maple syrup.

Serving Suggestions:

- Top with sliced bananas or berries for added freshness.

- Spread a thin layer of almond butter between the pancakes.

- Garnish with a sprinkle of chopped nuts like almonds or walnuts.

Sardine and Avocado Toast

Preparation Time: 10 minutes

Serves: 2

Ingredients:

- 1 can (3.75 oz) sardines in olive oil, drained
- 1 ripe avocado
- 4 slices whole-grain bread, toasted
- 1 lemon, juiced
- Salt and pepper to taste
- Red pepper flakes for a hint of spice (optional)
- Fresh parsley for garnish (optional)

Nutritional Information: Calories: 320kcal | Protein: 15g | Carbohydrates: 25g | Fat: 18g | Fiber: 10g

Instructions:

1. Use a fork to mash the ripe avocado in a bowl until it turns smooth.
2. Add lemon juice, salt, and pepper to the mashed avocado, mixing well.
3. Spread the avocado mixture evenly on each slice of toasted whole-grain bread.
4. Place sardines on top of the avocado spread, distributing them evenly.

5. If desired, sprinkle red pepper flakes for a touch of spice.

6. Sprinkle fresh parsley on top for a pop of color.

7. Serve immediately.

Serving Suggestions:

- Add a poached or fried egg on top for extra protein.

- Drizzle with a touch of olive oil for richness.

- Serve with a side of mixed greens dressed in a lemon vinaigrette.

Coconut Flour Banana Muffins

Preparation Time: 25 minutes

Serves: 12

Ingredients:

- 3 ripe bananas, mashed

- 4 large eggs

- 1/4 cup coconut oil, melted

- 1/4 cup honey or maple syrup

- 1 teaspoon vanilla extract

- 1/2 cup coconut flour

- 1/2 teaspoon baking soda

- 1/4 teaspoon salt
- 1/2 teaspoon cinnamon
- Chopped nuts for topping (optional)

Nutritional Information: Calories: 120kcal | Protein: 2g | Carbohydrates: 15g | Fat: 6g | Fiber: 3g

Instructions:

1. Preheat the oven to 350°F (175°C). Set up a muffin tin with paper liners.
2. In a large bowl, whisk together mashed bananas, eggs, melted coconut oil, honey or maple syrup, and vanilla extract.
3. In a separate bowl, combine coconut flour, baking soda, salt, and cinnamon.
4. Mix the dry ingredients into the wet ingredients slowly until a well-combined mixture forms.
5. Using a spoon, fill each cup of the prepared muffin tin about two-thirds full with the batter.
6. If desired, sprinkle chopped nuts on top of each muffin.
7. Bake until a toothpick inserted into the center is clean, which should take 18-20 minutes.

8. After 5 minutes of cooling in the tin, transfer the muffins to a wire rack to cool completely.

Serving Suggestions:

- Spread a thin layer of almond butter on a split muffin for added flavor.
- Enjoy with a cup of herbal tea or coffee in the morning.

Lox and Cucumber Toast

Preparation Time: 15 minutes

Serves: 2

Ingredients:

- 4 slices whole-grain bread, toasted
- 4 oz smoked salmon (lox)
- 1/2 cucumber, thinly sliced
- 4 oz cream cheese, softened
- 1 tablespoon capers, drained
- Fresh dill for garnish
- Lemon wedges for serving

Nutritional Information: Calories: 300kcal | Protein: 15g | Carbohydrates: 25g | Fat: 15g | Fiber: 5g

Instructions:

1. Toast the whole-grain bread slices until golden brown.
2. Spread a generous layer of softened cream cheese on each slice.
3. Arrange thinly sliced cucumber on top of the cream cheese.
4. Lay smoked salmon (lox) over the cucumber slices.
5. Sprinkle capers evenly over the salmon.
6. Garnish with fresh dill for added flavor.
7. Serve with lemon wedges on the side.

Serving Suggestions:

- Add a sprinkle of black pepper for extra zest.
- Top with finely chopped red onion for added crunch.
- Enjoy with a side of mixed greens dressed in a light vinaigrette.

CHAPTER 3

Lunch Recipes for Blood Type O

Chicken and Vegetable Curry with Coconut Milk and Rice

Preparation Time: 30 minutes

Serves: 4

Ingredients:

- 1 lb boneless, skinless chicken breast, cubed
- 1 can (14 oz) coconut milk
- 2 cups mixed vegetables (bell peppers, carrots, snap peas)
- 1 onion, finely chopped
- 3 cloves garlic, minced
- 1 tablespoon curry powder
- 1 teaspoon turmeric
- 1 teaspoon cumin
- 1 cup basmati rice
- 2 tablespoons olive oil
- Salt and pepper to taste
- Fresh cilantro for garnish (optional)

Nutritional Information: Calories: 450kcal | Protein: 25g | Carbohydrates: 35g | Fat: 20g | Fiber: 4g

Instructions:

1. Cook basmati rice according to package instructions.
2. Heat olive oil in a large skillet set to medium heat.
3. Add chopped onions and sauté until translucent.
4. Add minced garlic and cook for an additional 1-2 minutes until fragrant.
5. Add cubed chicken to the skillet and cook until browned on all sides.
6. Sprinkle curry powder, turmeric, and cumin over the chicken, stirring to coat evenly.
7. Pour in coconut milk and bring the mixture to a simmer.
8. Add mixed vegetables to the skillet and cook until they are tender-crisp.
9. Season with salt and pepper to taste.
10. Serve the curry over a bed of cooked basmati rice.

11. Garnish with fresh cilantro if desired.

Serving Suggestions:

- Pair with a side of steamed broccoli for added greens.
- Enjoy with a squeeze of fresh lime for a citrusy kick.
- Serve alongside a small portion of sliced avocado.

Kale and Avocado Salad with Walnuts and Lemon Dressing

Preparation Time: 15 minutes

Serves: 2

Ingredients:

- 4 cups of kale with the stems removed, and the leaves chopped
- 1 ripe avocado, diced
- 1/2 cup walnuts, chopped
- 1/4 cup feta cheese, crumbled
- 1 lemon, juiced
- 3 tablespoons olive oil
- 1 teaspoon Dijon mustard

- 1 teaspoon honey

- Salt and pepper to taste

Nutritional Information: Calories: 380kcal | Protein: 10g | Carbohydrates: 20g | Fat: 30g | Fiber: 7g

Instructions:

1. In a large salad bowl, combine chopped kale, diced avocado, chopped walnuts, and crumbled feta cheese.
2. In a small bowl, whisk together lemon juice, olive oil, Dijon mustard, honey, salt, and pepper to create the dressing.
3. Pour the dressing over the salad and toss until the ingredients are well coated.
4. Allow the salad to sit for a few minutes to let the flavors meld.
5. Serve immediately.

Serving Suggestions:

- Top with grilled chicken or shrimp for an added protein boost.
- Add a handful of cherry tomatoes for extra freshness.

- Enjoy with a side of whole-grain bread or a quinoa bowl.

Mediterranean Steak Salad

Preparation Time: 25 minutes

Serves: 2

Ingredients:

- 1 lb sirloin steak
- 4 cups mixed greens (spinach, arugula, romaine)
- 1 cup cherry tomatoes, halved
- 1 cucumber, sliced
- 1/2 red onion, thinly sliced
- 1/4 cup Kalamata olives, pitted
- 1/4 cup feta cheese, crumbled
- 2 tablespoons olive oil
- 1 tablespoon red wine vinegar
- 1 teaspoon dried oregano
- Salt and pepper to taste

Nutritional Information: Calories: 480kcal | Protein: 40g | Carbohydrates: 15g | Fat: 30g | Fiber: 5g

Instructions:

1. Season the sirloin steak with salt, pepper, and dried oregano.
2. Grill the steak to your preferred doneness, then let it rest before slicing.
3. In a large salad bowl, combine mixed greens, cherry tomatoes, cucumber, red onion, Kalamata olives, and crumbled feta cheese.
4. Whisk together olive oil and red wine vinegar in a small bowl to make the dressing.
5. Drizzle the dressing over the salad and toss until well combined.
6. Slice the grilled steak and arrange the slices on top of the salad.
7. Serve immediately.

Serving Suggestions:

- Garnish with chopped fresh parsley to add a burst of flavor.
- Add a side of hummus or tzatziki for a Mediterranean dip.
- Enjoy with a slice of whole-grain bread or pita.

Quinoa and Vegetable Stir-Fry

Preparation Time: 20 minutes

Serves: 4

Ingredients:

- 1 cup quinoa, uncooked
- 2 cups broccoli florets
- 1 red bell pepper, sliced
- 1 yellow bell pepper, sliced
- 1 carrot, julienned
- 1 zucchini, sliced
- 3 tablespoons tamari sauce
- 2 tablespoons sesame oil
- 1 tablespoon olive oil
- 2 cloves garlic, minced
- 1 teaspoon ginger, grated
- Sesame seeds for garnish (optional)
- Green onions for garnish (optional)

Nutritional Information: Calories: 320kcal | Protein: 10g | Carbohydrates: 45g | Fat: 12g | Fiber: 8g

Instructions:

1. Rinse quinoa under cold water, then cook according to package instructions.
2. In a large wok or skillet, heat your olive oil on a medium-high heat.
3. Sauté minced grated ginger and garlic until they release their aroma.
4. Add broccoli, red and yellow bell peppers, julienned carrot, and sliced zucchini to the skillet. Stir-fry the vegetables for 4-5 minutes until they reach a crisp-tender state.
5. Push the vegetables to the side of the skillet, add a bit more oil if needed, and crack an egg into the skillet. Scramble the egg and integrate it with the vegetables.
6. Add cooked quinoa to the skillet, pouring tamari sauce and sesame oil over the mixture. Mix until thoroughly combined and heated through.
7. Add sesame seeds and green onions as garnish if you like.
8. Serve immediately.

Serving Suggestions:

- Enhance with grilled chicken or tofu for an extra protein boost.
- Drizzle with a bit of Sriracha for a spicy kick.
- Enjoy as a standalone dish or as a side with grilled fish.

Cauliflower Fried Rice with Shrimp

Preparation Time: 20 minutes

Serves: 2

Ingredients:

- 1 head cauliflower, grated
- 8 oz shrimp, peeled and deveined
- 1 cup mixed vegetables (peas, carrots, corn)
- 2 eggs, beaten
- 2 tablespoons soy sauce
- 1 tablespoon sesame oil
- 1 tablespoon olive oil
- 2 cloves garlic, minced
- 1 teaspoon ginger, grated
- Green onions for garnish (optional)
- Sesame seeds for garnish (optional)

Nutritional Information: Calories: 320kcal | Protein: 25g | Carbohydrates: 20g | Fat: 15g | Fiber: 8g

Instructions:

1. In a large wok or skillet, heat your olive oil on a medium-high heat.
2. Sauté minced grated ginger and garlic until they release their aroma.
3. Introduce shrimp to the skillet and cook until they become pink and opaque. Take the shrimp out of the skillet and place them aside.
4. In the same skillet, add beaten eggs and scramble until cooked. Remove eggs and set aside.
5. Add more oil if needed, then add grated cauliflower and mixed vegetables to the skillet. Stir-fry for 5-6 minutes until the cauliflower is tender.
6. Return the cooked shrimp and scrambled eggs to the skillet.

7. Pour soy sauce and sesame oil over the mixture, tossing until everything is well combined and heated through.

8. Optionally, top with chopped green onions and sesame seeds for garnish.

9. Serve immediately.

Serving Suggestions:

- Spice it up with a dash of hot sauce for an added kick.
- Top with fresh cilantro for a burst of flavor.
- Pair with a side of kimchi or pickled vegetables.

Turkey Lettuce Wraps

Preparation Time: 20 minutes

Serves: 4

Ingredients:

- 1 lb ground turkey
- 1 tablespoon olive oil
- 1 onion, finely chopped
- 2 cloves garlic, minced
- 1 tablespoon ginger, grated

- 1 red bell pepper, diced
- 1 carrot, julienned
- 1/4 cup hoisin sauce
- 2 tablespoons soy sauce
- 1 tablespoon rice vinegar
- 1 teaspoon sesame oil
- Bibb or iceberg lettuce leaves for wrapping
- Green onions for garnish (optional)
- Sesame seeds for garnish (optional)

Nutritional Information: Calories: 280kcal | Protein: 20g | Carbohydrates: 15g | Fat: 15g | Fiber: 3g

Instructions:

1. Heat olive oil in a large skillet set to medium heat.
2. Introduce grated ginger, chopped onion and minced garlic to the skillet. Sauté until the onion is translucent.
3. Place ground turkey in the skillet and cook until it turns brown.
4. Add diced red bell pepper and julienned carrot to the skillet. Continue stir-frying for an extra 3-

4 minutes until the vegetables reach a tender state.

5. Mix hoisin sauce, soy sauce, rice vinegar, and sesame oil together in a small bowl.
6. Pour the sauce over the turkey and vegetable mixture, tossing until well coated and heated through.
7. Spoon the turkey mixture into individual lettuce leaves, creating wraps.
8. Optionally, top with chopped green onions and sesame seeds for garnish.
9. Serve immediately.

Serving Suggestions:

- Top with a sprinkle of crushed peanuts for added crunch.
- Drizzle with Sriracha for those who enjoy a bit of heat.
- Enjoy with a side of pickled radishes or cucumber.

Salmon and Asparagus Foil Packets

Preparation Time: 25 minutes

Serves: 2

Ingredients:

- 2 salmon fillets
- 1 bunch asparagus, trimmed
- 1 lemon, thinly sliced
- 2 tablespoons olive oil
- 2 cloves garlic, minced
- 1 teaspoon Dijon mustard
- 1 teaspoon dried dill
- Salt and pepper to taste
- Fresh parsley for garnish (optional)

Nutritional Information: Calories: 350kcal | Protein: 30g | Carbohydrates: 10g | Fat: 20g | Fiber: 5g

Instructions:

1. Preheat the oven to 400°F (200°C).
2. Cut two large pieces of aluminum foil.

3. In a bowl, whisk together olive oil, minced garlic, Dijon mustard, dried dill, salt, and pepper.
4. Place a salmon fillet in the middle of each foil sheet.
5. Arrange trimmed asparagus around the salmon.
6. Drizzle the olive oil mixture over the salmon and asparagus.
7. Top each salmon fillet with lemon slices.
8. Fold the foil over the salmon and asparagus, sealing the edges to create a packet.
9. Set the foil packets on a baking sheet and bake in the preheated oven for 15-20 minutes or until the salmon is fully cooked.
10. Unfold the foil packets carefully, add a touch of fresh parsley if desired, and serve.

Serving Suggestions:

- Serve over a bed of quinoa or cauliflower rice.
- Enjoy with a side of mixed greens dressed in a light vinaigrette.

- Add a sprinkle of capers for an extra burst of flavor.

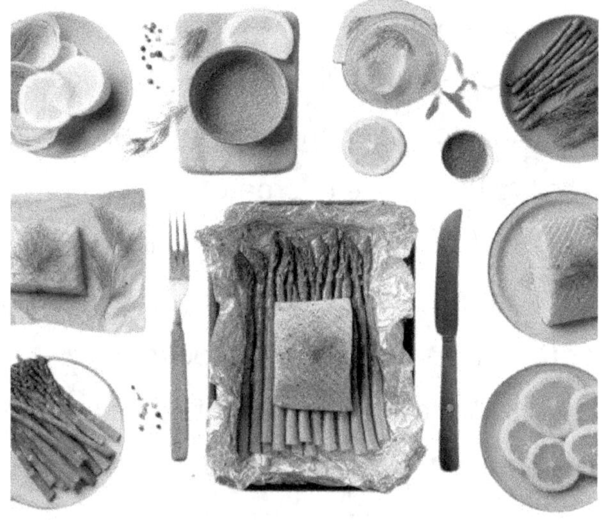

CHAPTER 4

Dinner Recipes for Blood Type O

Sweet Potato and Turkey Chili

Preparation Time: 30 minutes

Serves: 4

Ingredients:

- 1 lb ground turkey
- 2 sweet potatoes, peeled and diced
- 1 can (15 oz) of drained and rinsed kidney beans
- 1 can (15 oz) diced tomatoes
- 1 onion, finely chopped
- 3 cloves garlic, minced
- 2 tablespoons chili powder
- 1 teaspoon cumin
- 1 teaspoon paprika
- 1/2 teaspoon cinnamon
- 2 cups low-sodium chicken broth
- Salt and pepper to taste
- Avocado slices for garnish (optional)

- Fresh cilantro for garnish (optional)

Nutritional Information: Calories: 400kcal | Protein: 25g | Carbohydrates: 45g | Fat: 15g | Fiber: 10g

Instructions:

1. Heat up olive oil in a large pot over medium heat.
2. Add chopped onion and minced garlic, sautéing until the onion is translucent.
3. Add ground turkey to the pot and cook until browned.
4. Stir in chili powder, cumin, paprika, and cinnamon, ensuring the turkey is well coated.
5. Add diced sweet potatoes, kidney beans, diced tomatoes, and chicken broth to the pot.
6. Bring the mixture to a simmer and let it cook for 20-25 minutes or until the sweet potatoes are tender.
7. Season with salt and pepper to taste.
8. Serve the chili hot, garnished with avocado slices and fresh cilantro if desired.

- Top with a dollop of Greek yogurt for added creaminess.
- Enjoy with a side of whole-grain cornbread.
- Sprinkle with shredded cheddar cheese for an extra layer of flavor.

Eggplant and Tomato Bake

Preparation Time: 35 minutes

Serves: 4

Ingredients:

- 2 large eggplants, sliced
- 4 large tomatoes, sliced
- 1 cup mozzarella cheese, shredded
- 1/4 cup Parmesan cheese, grated
- 2 cloves garlic, minced
- 2 tablespoons olive oil
- 1 teaspoon dried oregano
- 1 teaspoon dried basil
- Salt and pepper to taste
- Fresh basil for garnish (optional)

Nutritional Information: Calories: 220kcal | Protein: 10g | Carbohydrates: 20g | Fat: 14g | Fiber: 8g

Instructions:

1. Preheat the oven to 375°F (190°C).
2. In a bowl, mix together olive oil, minced garlic, dried oregano, dried basil, salt, and pepper.
3. Brush both sides of eggplant slices with the olive oil mixture.
4. In a baking dish, layer sliced tomatoes and eggplant, alternating and slightly overlapping.
5. Sprinkle shredded mozzarella and grated Parmesan evenly over the layers.
6. Repeat the layering process until all the ingredients are used, finishing with a layer of cheese on top.
7. Bake until the cheese is melted and bubbly, which should take 25-30 minutes in the preheated oven.
8. Take it out of the oven and let it cool a bit before serving.
9. Garnish with fresh basil if desired.

Serving Suggestions:

- Serve as a side dish with grilled chicken or fish.

- Enjoy with a side of quinoa or couscous for a complete meal.
- Drizzle with balsamic glaze for added sweetness.

Cauliflower Pizza with Turkey Pepperoni

Preparation Time: 40 minutes

Serves: 2-4

Ingredients:

- 1 head cauliflower, grated
- 1 cup mozzarella cheese, shredded
- 1/4 cup Parmesan cheese, grated
- 1 egg
- 1 teaspoon dried oregano
- 1 teaspoon dried basil
- 1/2 teaspoon garlic powder
- 1/2 teaspoon onion powder
- Salt and pepper to taste
- 1/2 cup tomato sauce
- 1 cup turkey pepperoni slices
- 1/2 cup black olives, sliced
- 1/2 cup bell peppers, sliced

- Fresh basil for garnish (optional)

Nutritional Information: Calories: 280kcal | Protein: 18g | Carbohydrates: 15g | Fat: 16g | Fiber: 7g

Instructions:

1. Preheat the oven to 425°F (220°C).

2. Place grated cauliflower in a microwave-safe bowl and microwave for 5 minutes.

3. Allow the cauliflower to cool before transferring it to a clean kitchen towel. Squeeze out excess moisture.

4. In a bowl, combine cauliflower, mozzarella cheese, Parmesan cheese, egg, dried oregano, dried basil, garlic powder, onion powder, salt, and pepper. Mix until well combined.

5. Line a baking sheet with parchment paper and spread the cauliflower mixture into a thin, even circle, resembling a pizza crust.

6. Bake the crust in the preheated oven for 15-20 minutes or until golden brown.

7. Take the crust out of the oven and evenly spread tomato sauce over the surface.

8. Top with turkey pepperoni slices, black olives, and bell peppers.

9. Place the pizza back in the oven and bake for an extra 10-15 minutes, or until the cheese is melted and bubbling.

10. Garnish with fresh basil if desired.

Serving Suggestions:

- Enjoy this with a light salad or a side of mixed greens.
- Drizzle with olive oil for extra richness.
- Add a touch of spice by sprinkling with red pepper flakes.

Rice Porridge with Cinnamon and Nuts

Preparation Time: 40 minutes

Serves: 4

Ingredients:

- 1 cup brown rice
- 4 cups water
- 2 cups almond milk
- 1/4 cup honey or maple syrup
- 1 teaspoon ground cinnamon

- 1/2 teaspoon vanilla extract
- 1/2 cup mixed nuts (almonds, walnuts, pistachios), chopped
- Fresh berries for topping (optional)
- Coconut flakes for topping (optional)

Nutritional Information: Calories: 250kcal | Protein: 6g | Carbohydrates: 45g | Fat: 7g | Fiber: 4g

Instructions:

1. In a large pot, combine brown rice and water. Bring to a boil, then reduce heat to low and simmer, covered, for 30-35 minutes or until the rice is cooked and water is absorbed.
2. Stir in almond milk, honey or maple syrup, ground cinnamon, and vanilla extract.
3. Continue to cook over low heat, stirring occasionally, for an additional 10 minutes or until the porridge reaches your desired consistency.
4. Remove from the heat source and let it cool briefly before serving.
5. Divide the rice porridge into bowls and top with chopped mixed nuts.

6. If desired, garnish with fresh berries and coconut flakes.

Serving Suggestions:

- Drizzle with additional honey or maple syrup for sweetness.

- Add a splash of almond milk before serving for creaminess.

Venison and Mushroom Pie with Spelt Crust

Preparation Time: 1 hour

Serves: 6

Ingredients:

- 1 lb venison, cubed
- 2 cups mushrooms, sliced
- 1 onion, finely chopped
- 2 cloves garlic, minced
- 2 tablespoons olive oil
- 2 tablespoons spelt flour
- 1 cup beef or vegetable broth
- 1/2 cup red wine
- 1 teaspoon dried thyme

- Salt and pepper to taste
- 1 sheet spelt puff pastry
- 1 egg, beaten (for egg wash)
- Fresh parsley for garnish (optional)

Nutritional Information: Calories: 400kcal | Protein: 25g | Carbohydrates: 20g | Fat: 25g | Fiber: 4g

Instructions:

1. Preheat the oven to 375°F (190°C).
2. Heat olive oil in a large skillet set to medium heat.
3. Add chopped onion and minced garlic, sautéing until the onion is translucent.
4. Add cubed venison to the skillet and brown on all sides.
5. Sprinkle spelt flour over the venison and stir to coat evenly.
6. Pour in red wine and beef or vegetable broth, stirring to combine.
7. Add sliced mushrooms, dried thyme, salt, and pepper to the skillet. Simmer for 15-20 minutes or until the venison is tender and the mixture has thickened.

8. Transfer the venison and mushroom filling to a pie dish.

9. Roll out the spelt puff pastry sheet and place it over the filling, trimming any excess.

10. Coat the pastry with beaten egg for a golden appearance.

11. Place in the preheated oven and bake for 25-30 minutes or until the pastry is puffed up and turns golden.

12. Garnish with fresh parsley if desired.

Serving Suggestions:

- Pair it with a side of steamed vegetables or a fresh green salad.
- Enjoy with a glass of red wine for a delightful pairing.
- Serve as a hearty dinner on colder evenings.

Vegetable and Tofu Curry

Preparation Time: 35 minutes

Serves: 4

Ingredients:

- 1 block firm tofu, cubed
- 2 cups mixed vegetables (broccoli, bell peppers, carrots, peas)
- 1 can (14 oz) coconut milk
- 1 onion, finely chopped
- 3 cloves garlic, minced
- 1 tablespoon red curry paste
- 1 teaspoon turmeric
- 1 teaspoon cumin
- 1 teaspoon coriander
- 1 tablespoon soy sauce
- 1 tablespoon olive oil
- Fresh cilantro for garnish (optional)
- Lime wedges for serving

Nutritional Information: Calories: 320kcal | Protein: 15g | Carbohydrates: 20g | Fat: 22g | Fiber: 6g

Instructions:

1. Heat olive oil in a large skillet set to medium heat.
2. Add chopped onion and minced garlic, sautéing until the onion is translucent.
3. Place cubed tofu into the skillet and cook until it turns golden brown on all sides.
4. Stir in red curry paste, turmeric, cumin, and coriander, ensuring the tofu is well coated.
5. Add mixed vegetables to the skillet and sauté for 5-7 minutes until they are tender-crisp.
6. Pour in coconut milk and soy sauce, stirring to combine. Simmer for an additional 10 minutes.
7. Season with salt and pepper to taste.
8. Garnish with fresh cilantro if desired.
9. Serve the vegetable and tofu curry over a bed of cooked brown rice or quinoa.
10. Squeeze lime wedges over the curry before serving.

Serving Suggestions:

- Enjoy with naan bread or whole-grain roti.
- Garnish with chopped peanuts or cashews to introduce a satisfying crunch.

Mushroom Risotto with Parmesan Cheese and Parsley

Preparation Time: 40 minutes

Serves: 4

Ingredients:

- 2 cups Arborio rice
- 1 lb mushrooms, sliced
- 1 onion, finely chopped
- 2 cloves garlic, minced
- 1/2 cup dry white wine
- 6 cups vegetable or chicken broth, kept warm
- 1/2 cup Parmesan cheese, grated
- 2 tablespoons olive oil
- 2 tablespoons butter
- Fresh parsley, chopped, for garnish
- Salt and pepper to taste

Nutritional Information: Calories: 400kcal | Protein: 10g | Carbohydrates: 70g | Fat: 10g | Fiber: 3g

Instructions:

1. In a large skillet or wide saucepan, heat olive oil over medium heat.
2. Add chopped onion and cook until translucent.
3. Add minced garlic and sliced mushrooms, sautéing until the mushrooms are browned.
4. Stir in Arborio rice and cook for 1-2 minutes until the rice is lightly toasted.
5. Pour in the white wine, stirring until it is mostly absorbed by the rice.
6. Gradually incorporate the warm broth, one ladleful at a time, stirring consistently. Allow the liquid to be mostly absorbed before adding the next ladleful.
7. Continue with the process until the rice becomes creamy and reaches al dente, typically in about 18-20 minutes.

8. Stir in grated Parmesan cheese and butter, mixing until well combined.

9. Season with salt and pepper to taste.

10. Garnish with chopped fresh parsley before serving.

Serving Suggestions:

- Serve as a main dish or a side alongside grilled chicken or fish.

- Top with additional Parmesan cheese for extra richness.

- Pair with a crisp green salad for a well-rounded meal.

CHAPTER 5

Desserts and Snacks Recipes for Blood Type O

Frozen Banana "Ice Cream"

Preparation Time: 10 minutes (plus freezing time)

Serves: 2

Ingredients:

- 2 ripe bananas, peeled and sliced
- 1 tablespoon almond butter
- 1 teaspoon vanilla extract
- 2 tablespoons unsweetened almond milk
- Toppings of choice: chopped nuts, shredded coconut, dark chocolate chips

Nutritional Information: Calories: 150kcal | Protein: 2g | Carbohydrates: 30g | Fat: 5g | Fiber: 4g

Instructions:

1. Arrange the banana slices on a parchment-lined tray and freeze until solid (about 2 hours or overnight).

2. In a food processor, combine the frozen banana slices, almond butter, vanilla extract, and almond milk.

3. Blend and scrape the sides as needed until it becomes creamy and smooth.

4. Transfer the "ice cream" to a bowl and swirl in your favorite toppings.

5. Serve immediately for a soft-serve consistency or freeze for an additional 30 minutes for a firmer texture.

Serving Suggestions:

- Top with a sprinkle of chopped nuts for added crunch.
- Drizzle with a bit of honey or maple syrup for sweetness.
- Garnish with a few dark chocolate chips for a decadent touch.

Dark Chocolate-Dipped Strawberries

Preparation Time: 20 minutes

Serves: 4

Ingredients:

- 1 pint fresh strawberries, washed and dried
- 4 oz dark chocolate, chopped
- 1 teaspoon coconut oil
- Toppings of choice: chopped nuts, shredded coconut, sea salt

Nutritional Information: Calories: 100kcal | Protein: 1g | Carbohydrates: 10g | Fat: 7g | Fiber: 3g

Instructions:

1. In a heatproof bowl, melt the dark chocolate and coconut oil together. You can use a double boiler or microwave in 20-second intervals, stirring until smooth.
2. Dip each strawberry by the stem into the melted chocolate, swirling to ensure an even coating.

3. Allow excess chocolate to drip off, then place the dipped strawberry on a parchment-lined tray.

4. Repeat with the remaining strawberries.

5. Optional: Sprinkle your choice of toppings over the chocolate-dipped strawberries while the chocolate is still wet.

6. Refrigerate the strawberries for at least 15 minutes or until the chocolate is set.

7. Serve chilled.

Serving Suggestions:

- Drizzle with a bit of melted white chocolate for a decorative touch.
- Garnish with a sprinkle of sea salt for a sweet and savory contrast.
- Enjoy as a light and elegant dessert or snack.

Peanut Butter Cookies

Preparation Time: 20 minutes

Serves: 12 cookies

Ingredients:

- 1 cup almond flour
- 1/2 cup peanut butter
- 1/4 cup coconut oil, melted
- 1/4 cup honey or maple syrup
- 1 teaspoon vanilla extract
- 1/2 teaspoon baking soda
- 1/4 teaspoon salt
- Toppings of choice: crushed peanuts, dark chocolate drizzle

Nutritional Information: Calories: 150kcal | Protein: 4g | Carbohydrates: 8g | Fat: 12g | Fiber: 2g

Instructions:

1. Preheat your oven to 350°F (180°C) and prepare a baking sheet by lining it with parchment paper.
2. In a bowl, mix together almond flour, peanut butter, melted coconut oil, honey or maple syrup, vanilla extract, baking soda, and salt until well combined.
3. Use a tablespoon to scoop portions of the dough, then roll them into balls. Place them on the prepared baking sheet.

4. Flatten each cookie with a fork, creating a crisscross pattern on the top.

5. Optional: Sprinkle crushed peanuts over the cookies before baking.

6. Place in the preheated oven and bake for 10-12 minutes or until the edges turn golden brown.

7. Cool the cookies on the baking sheet for 5 minutes, then move them to a wire rack for complete cooling.

8. Optional: Drizzle with melted dark chocolate for extra indulgence.

Serving Suggestions:

- Enjoy with a glass of almond milk for a classic combination.
- Pair with a scoop of vanilla or banana "ice cream."
- Store in an airtight container for a delicious grab-and-go snack.

Roasted Chickpeas

Preparation Time: 40 minutes

Serves: 4

Ingredients:

- 2 cans (15 oz each) chickpeas, drained and rinsed
- 2 tablespoons olive oil
- 1 teaspoon smoked paprika
- 1/2 teaspoon cumin
- 1/2 teaspoon garlic powder
- 1/4 teaspoon cayenne pepper (adjust to taste)
- Salt to taste

Nutritional Information: Calories: 180kcal | Protein: 6g | Carbohydrates: 23g | Fat: 7g | Fiber: 6g

Instructions:

1. Preheat your oven to 400°F (200°C) and prepare a baking sheet by lining it with parchment paper.
2. Rinse and thoroughly dry chickpeas with a kitchen towel.

3. In a bowl, toss chickpeas with olive oil, smoked paprika, cumin, garlic powder, cayenne pepper, and salt until well coated.
4. Evenly spread the seasoned chickpeas on the prepared baking sheet in a single layer.
5. Bake in the preheated oven for 30-35 minutes or until the chickpeas are golden and crispy, shaking the pan halfway through.
6. Take them out of the oven and let them cool a bit before serving.

Serving Suggestions:

- Enjoy as a crunchy snack on its own.
- Sprinkle over salads or soups for added texture.
- Serve alongside your favorite dip for a flavorful appetizer.

Edamame with Sea Salt

Preparation Time: 10 minutes

Serves: 4

Ingredients:

- 2 cups frozen edamame, thawed
- 1 tablespoon olive oil
- Sea salt to taste

Nutritional Information: Calories: 120kcal | Protein: 9g | Carbohydrates: 8g | Fat: 6g | Fiber: 4g

Instructions:

1. Bring a pot of water to boil and cook the edamame according to package instructions. Drain and set aside.
2. Over medium heat, heat your olive oil in a skillet.
3. Add the cooked edamame to the skillet, stirring to coat with the oil.
4. Sauté for 5-7 minutes or until the edamame is slightly crispy.
5. Sprinkle with sea salt to taste, tossing to ensure even seasoning.

6. Serve warm.

Serving Suggestions:

- Enjoy as a protein-packed snack on its own.
- Sprinkle with sesame seeds for added crunch and flavor.

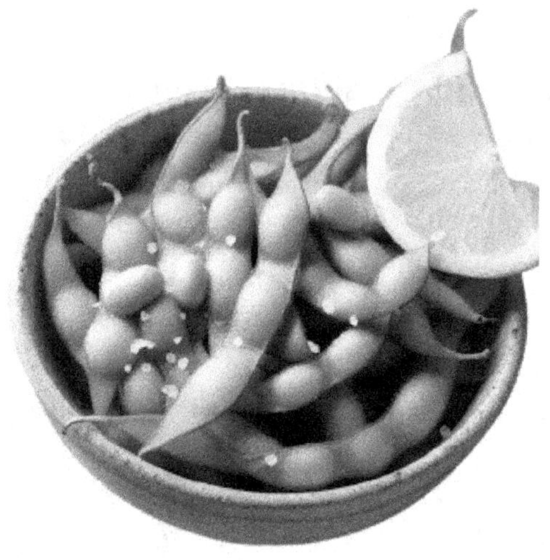

CHAPTER 6

Beverages and Smoothies for Blood Type O

Berry Citrus Sparkling Water

Preparation Time: 5 minutes

Serves: 2

Ingredients:

- 1 cup mixed berries (strawberries, blueberries, raspberries)
- 1 orange, thinly sliced
- 1 lemon, thinly sliced
- 2 sprigs fresh mint
- Ice cubes
- 2 cups sparkling water

Nutritional Information: Calories: 20kcal | Protein: 1g | Carbohydrates: 5g | Fiber: 2g | Sugar: 2g

Instructions:

1. In a pitcher, combine mixed berries, orange slices, lemon slices, and fresh mint.

2. Fill the pitcher with ice cubes.

3. Pour the sparkling water into the pitcher with the ingredients.

4. Stir gently to combine the flavors.

5. Serve the Berry Citrus Sparkling Water in glasses, ensuring each serving has a variety of berries and citrus slices.

Serving Suggestions:

- Enhance the freshness by garnishing with extra mint leaves.
- Customize sweetness by adding a drizzle of honey if desired.
- Enjoy as a hydrating and flavorful alternative to sugary sodas.

Iced Peppermint Tea

Preparation Time: 15 minutes (plus chilling time)

Serves: 4

Ingredients:

- 4 peppermint tea bags
- 4 cups boiling water
- 1-2 tablespoons honey or maple syrup (optional)

- Fresh mint leaves for garnish

- Ice cubes

Nutritional Information: Calories: 5kcal | Protein: 0g | Carbohydrates: 1g | Fat: 0g | Sugar: 0g

Instructions:

1. Place peppermint tea bags in a heatproof pitcher.
2. Pour boiling water over the tea bags and steep for 5-7 minutes.
3. Optional: Add honey or maple syrup to the tea for sweetness, stirring until dissolved.
4. Take out the tea bags and allow the tea to cool down to room temperature.
5. Refrigerate the tea for at least 2 hours or until chilled.
6. Fill glasses with ice cubes.
7. Pour the chilled peppermint tea over the ice in each glass.
8. Garnish with fresh mint leaves.

Serving Suggestions:

- Serve with a wedge of lemon for added citrusy freshness.

- Pair with a slice of cucumber or a sprig of basil for a unique twist.
- Enjoy as a soothing and cooling beverage on a warm day.

Tropical Green Smoothie

Preparation Time: 10 minutes

Serves: 2

Ingredients:

- 1 cup fresh spinach leaves
- 1/2 cup pineapple chunks (fresh or frozen)
- 1/2 cup mango chunks (fresh or frozen)
- 1 banana
- 1 cup coconut water
- 1 tablespoon chia seeds (optional)
- Ice cubes

Nutritional Information: Calories: 150kcal | Protein: 3g | Carbohydrates: 35g | Fat: 1g | Fiber: 6g

Instructions:

1. In a blender, combine fresh spinach leaves, pineapple chunks, mango chunks, banana, and coconut water.

2. Optional: Add chia seeds for an extra nutritional boost.

3. Blend until smooth and creamy.

4. Add ice cubes and blend once more until the smoothie reaches the consistency you desire.

5. Transfer the Tropical Green Smoothie into glasses and serve right away.

Serving Suggestions:

- Garnish with a slice of pineapple or a sprinkle of chia seeds for texture.

- Customize sweetness by adding a touch of honey or agave syrup if desired.

- Enjoy as a nutrient-packed breakfast or a refreshing afternoon pick-me-up.

Cucumber and Celery Refresher

Preparation Time: 10 minutes

Serves: 2

Ingredients:

- 1 cucumber, peeled and sliced

- 2 celery stalks, chopped

- 1/2 lemon, juiced
- 1 tablespoon fresh ginger, grated
- 1 tablespoon honey or agave syrup
- 2 cups cold water
- Ice cubes

Nutritional Information: Calories: 30kcal | Protein: 1g | Carbohydrates: 8g | Fat: 0g | Fiber: 2g

Instructions:

1. In a blender, combine cucumber slices, chopped celery, lemon juice, grated ginger, and honey or agave syrup.
2. Add cold water to the blender.
3. Blend the ingredients until smooth.
4. Strain the mixture using a fine mesh sieve or cheesecloth to remove pulp, if desired.
5. Fill glasses with ice cubes.
6. Pour the Cucumber and Celery Refresher over the ice in each glass.
7. Stir gently before serving.

Serving Suggestions:

- Garnish with a cucumber slice or a celery stalk for a decorative touch.
- Serve with a sprig of mint for added freshness.
- Enjoy as a hydrating and revitalizing drink.

Watermelon Lime Agua Fresca

Preparation Time: 15 minutes

Serves: 4

Ingredients:

- 4 cups fresh watermelon, cubed
- 2 limes, juiced
- 2 tablespoons of agave syrup or honey (adjust to your taste)
- 4 cups cold water
- Mint leaves for garnish
- Ice cubes

Nutritional Information: Calories: 40kcal | Protein: 1g | Carbohydrates: 10g | Fat: 0g | Fiber: 1g

Instructions:

1. In a blender, combine fresh watermelon cubes and lime juice.
2. Blend until smooth.
3. Strain the watermelon-lime mixture using a fine mesh sieve to remove pulp, if desired.
4. In a pitcher, mix the strained watermelon-lime juice with honey or agave syrup.
5. Add cold water to the pitcher and stir until well combined.
6. Fill glasses with ice cubes.
7. Pour the Watermelon Lime Agua Fresca over the ice in each glass.
8. Garnish with mint leaves.

Serving Suggestions:

- Rim glasses with a touch of salt for a sweet and salty contrast.
- Add a hint of sparkling water for a bubbly effect.
- Enjoy as a refreshing and hydrating beverage on a hot day.

CHAPTER 7

30 Days Meal Plan For Blood Type O

Please note that the provided meal plan is a sample and should not be interpreted as a recommendation to consume all the listed recipes in a single day.

The purpose of this meal plan is to offer inspiration and guidance for healthy meal preparation. Feel free to customize this plan further to suit your preferences and dietary requirements.

Day 1:

- *Breakfast:* Beef and Vegetable Stir-Fry with Buckwheat Noodles
- *Lunch:* Chicken and Vegetable Curry with Coconut Milk and Rice
- *Dinner:* Sweet Potato and Turkey Chili
- *Dessert/Snack:* Roasted Chickpeas
- *Beverage:* Cucumber and Celery Refresher

Day 2:

- *Breakfast:* Buckwheat Pancakes with Berry Compote
- *Lunch:* Kale and Avocado Salad with Walnuts and Lemon Dressing
- *Dinner:* Eggplant and Tomato Bake
- *Dessert/Snack:* Dark Chocolate-Dipped Strawberries
- *Beverage:* Tropical Green Smoothie

Day 3:

- *Breakfast:* Broccoli and Feta Frittata
- *Lunch:* Mediterranean Steak Salad
- *Dinner:* Cauliflower Pizza with Turkey Pepperoni
- *Dessert/Snack:* Edamame with Sea Salt
- *Beverage:* Watermelon Lime Agua Fresca

Day 4:

- *Breakfast:* Almond Flour Pancakes
- *Lunch:* Quinoa and Vegetable Stir-Fry
- *Dinner:* Rice Porridge with Cinnamon and Nuts
- *Dessert/Snack:* Peanut Butter Cookies

- *Beverage:* Iced Peppermint Tea

Day 5:

- *Breakfast:* Sardine and Avocado Toast
- *Lunch:* Cauliflower Fried Rice with Shrimp
- *Dinner:* Venison and Mushroom Pie with Spelt Crust
- *Dessert/Snack:* Frozen Banana "Ice Cream"
- *Beverage:* Berry Citrus Sparkling Water

Day 6:

- *Breakfast:* Coconut Flour Banana Muffins
- *Lunch:* Turkey Lettuce Wraps
- *Dinner:* Vegetable and Tofu Curry
- *Dessert/Snack:* Dark Chocolate-Dipped Strawberries
- *Beverage:* Iced Peppermint Tea

Day 7:

- *Breakfast:* Lox and Cucumber Toast
- *Lunch:* Salmon and Asparagus Foil Packets
- *Dinner:* Mushroom Risotto with Parmesan Cheese and Parsley

- *Dessert/Snack:* Roasted Chickpeas
- *Beverage:* Berry Citrus Sparkling Water

Day 8:

- *Breakfast:* Buckwheat Pancakes with Berry Compote
- *Lunch:* Chicken and Vegetable Curry with Coconut Milk and Rice
- *Dinner:* Sweet Potato and Turkey Chili
- *Dessert/Snack:* Peanut Butter Cookies
- *Beverage:* Tropical Green Smoothie

Day 9:

- *Breakfast:* Broccoli and Feta Frittata
- *Lunch:* Kale and Avocado Salad with Walnuts and Lemon Dressing
- *Dinner:* Eggplant and Tomato Bake
- *Dessert/Snack:* Roasted Chickpeas
- *Beverage:* Cucumber and Celery Refresher

Day 10:

- *Breakfast:* Almond Flour Pancakes
- *Lunch:* Mediterranean Steak Salad

- *Dinner:* Cauliflower Pizza with Turkey Pepperoni
- *Dessert/Snack:* Edamame with Sea Salt
- *Beverage:* Watermelon Lime Agua Fresca

Day 11:

- *Breakfast:* Sardine and Avocado Toast
- *Lunch:* Quinoa and Vegetable Stir-Fry
- *Dinner:* Rice Porridge with Cinnamon and Nuts
- *Dessert/Snack:* Peanut Butter Cookies
- *Beverage:* Iced Peppermint Tea

Day 12:

- *Breakfast:* Coconut Flour Banana Muffins
- *Lunch:* Cauliflower Fried Rice with Shrimp
- *Dinner:* Venison and Mushroom Pie with Spelt Crust
- *Dessert/Snack:* Frozen Banana "Ice Cream"
- *Beverage:* Berry Citrus Sparkling Water

Day 13:

- *Breakfast:* Lox and Cucumber Toast
- *Lunch:* Turkey Lettuce Wraps
- *Dinner:* Vegetable and Tofu Curry

- *Dessert/Snack:* Dark Chocolate-Dipped Strawberries
- *Beverage:* Iced Peppermint Tea

Day 14:

- *Breakfast:* Buckwheat Pancakes with Berry Compote
- *Lunch:* Salmon and Asparagus Foil Packets
- *Dinner:* Mushroom Risotto with Parmesan Cheese and Parsley
- *Dessert/Snack:* Roasted Chickpeas
- *Beverage:* Watermelon Lime Agua Fresca

Day 15:

- *Breakfast:* Beef and Vegetable Stir-Fry with Buckwheat Noodles
- *Lunch:* Chicken and Vegetable Curry with Coconut Milk and Rice
- *Dinner:* Sweet Potato and Turkey Chili

- *Dessert/Snack:* Dark Chocolate-Dipped Strawberries
- *Beverage:* Iced Peppermint Tea

Day 16:

- *Breakfast:* Buckwheat Pancakes with Berry Compote
- *Lunch:* Kale and Avocado Salad with Walnuts and Lemon Dressing
- *Dinner:* Eggplant and Tomato Bake
- *Dessert/Snack:* Peanut Butter Cookies
- *Beverage:* Tropical Green Smoothie

Day 17:

- *Breakfast:* Broccoli and Feta Frittata
- *Lunch:* Mediterranean Steak Salad

- *Dinner:* Cauliflower Pizza with Turkey Pepperoni
- *Dessert/Snack:* Edamame with Sea Salt
- *Beverage:* Watermelon Lime Agua Fresca

Day 18:

- *Breakfast:* Almond Flour Pancakes
- *Lunch:* Quinoa and Vegetable Stir-Fry
- *Dinner:* Rice Porridge with Cinnamon and Nuts
- *Dessert/Snack:* Roasted Chickpeas
- *Beverage:* Iced Peppermint Tea

Day 19:

- *Breakfast:* Sardine and Avocado Toast
- *Lunch:* Cauliflower Fried Rice with Shrimp
- *Dinner:* Venison and Mushroom Pie with Spelt Crust
- *Dessert/Snack:* Frozen Banana "Ice Cream"
- *Beverage:* Berry Citrus Sparkling Water

Day 20:

- *Breakfast:* Coconut Flour Banana Muffins
- *Lunch:* Turkey Lettuce Wraps
- *Dinner:* Vegetable and Tofu Curry
- *Dessert/Snack:* Dark Chocolate-Dipped Strawberries
- *Beverage:* Iced Peppermint Tea

Day 21:

- *Breakfast:* Lox and Cucumber Toast
- *Lunch:* Salmon and Asparagus Foil Packets
- *Dinner:* Mushroom Risotto with Parmesan Cheese and Parsley
- *Dessert/Snack:* Roasted Chickpeas
- *Beverage:* Watermelon Lime Agua Fresca

Day 22:

- *Breakfast:* Beef and Vegetable Stir-Fry with Buckwheat Noodles
- *Lunch:* Chicken and Vegetable Curry with Coconut Milk and Rice
- *Dinner:* Sweet Potato and Turkey Chili

- *Dessert/Snack:* Peanut Butter Cookies
- *Beverage:* Tropical Green Smoothie

Day 23:

- *Breakfast:* Buckwheat Pancakes with Berry Compote
- *Lunch:* Kale and Avocado Salad with Walnuts and Lemon Dressing
- *Dinner:* Eggplant and Tomato Bake
- *Dessert/Snack:* Dark Chocolate-Dipped Strawberries
- *Beverage:* Cucumber and Celery Refresher

Day 24:

- *Breakfast:* Broccoli and Feta Frittata
- *Lunch:* Mediterranean Steak Salad
- *Dinner:* Cauliflower Pizza with Turkey Pepperoni
- *Dessert/Snack:* Edamame with Sea Salt
- *Beverage:* Berry Citrus Sparkling Water

Day 25:

- *Breakfast:* Almond Flour Pancakes
- *Lunch:* Quinoa and Vegetable Stir-Fry
- *Dinner:* Rice Porridge with Cinnamon and Nuts
- *Dessert/Snack:* Roasted Chickpeas
- *Beverage:* Tropical Green Smoothie

Day 26:

- *Breakfast:* Sardine and Avocado Toast
- *Lunch:* Cauliflower Fried Rice with Shrimp
- *Dinner:* Venison and Mushroom Pie with Spelt Crust
- *Dessert/Snack:* Frozen Banana "Ice Cream"
- *Beverage:* Watermelon Lime Agua Fresca

Day 27:

- *Breakfast:* Coconut Flour Banana Muffins
- *Lunch:* Turkey Lettuce Wraps
- *Dinner:* Vegetable and Tofu Curry
- *Dessert/Snack:* Dark Chocolate-Dipped Strawberries

- *Beverage:* Iced Peppermint Tea

Day 28:

- *Breakfast:* Lox and Cucumber Toast
- *Lunch:* Salmon and Asparagus Foil Packets
- *Dinner:* Mushroom Risotto with Parmesan Cheese and Parsley
- *Dessert/Snack:* Roasted Chickpeas
- *Beverage:* Berry Citrus Sparkling Water

Day 29:

- *Breakfast:* Beef and Vegetable Stir-Fry with Buckwheat Noodles
- *Lunch:* Chicken and Vegetable Curry with Coconut Milk and Rice
- *Dinner:* Sweet Potato and Turkey Chili
- *Dessert/Snack:* Dark Chocolate-Dipped Strawberries
- *Beverage:* Iced Peppermint Tea

Day 30:

- *Breakfast:* Buckwheat Pancakes with Berry Compote

- *Lunch:* Kale and Avocado Salad with Walnuts and Lemon Dressing
- *Dinner:* Eggplant and Tomato Bake
- *Dessert/Snack:* Peanut Butter Cookies
- *Beverage:* Watermelon Lime Agua Fresca

CHAPTER 8

Conclusion

Congratulations on completing this culinary exploration tailored for Blood Type O individuals! As you close the pages of "Blood Type O Diet Recipes for Beginners," I hope you find yourself not just at the end of a cookbook but at the beginning of a vibrant and nourishing lifestyle.

In our journey together, we've delved into the intricacies of the Blood Type O diet, unlocking the secrets of foods that harmonize with your body's unique needs.

From the bustling aisles of the grocery store to the sizzling pans in your kitchen, you've gained insights into the powerful impact of selecting the right ingredients.

This cookbook isn't just a collection of recipes; it's a guide to transforming your relationship with food. We've discovered the art of crafting delicious meals that align with the Blood Type O principles—meals that not only tantalize your taste buds but also contribute to your overall well-being.

Beyond the recipes, this journey is about finding joy in the kitchen, exploring new tastes, and understanding the profound connection between what you eat and how you feel. It's about making informed choices that reflect your commitment to a healthier, more energized life.

As you embark on the continuation of your Blood Type O journey, remember that this is a flexible path. Feel free to experiment, tweak, and personalize these recipes to suit your taste preferences and dietary needs.

The goal is not perfection but progress—a journey toward optimal well-being that unfolds one delicious meal at a time.

May this cookbook be a constant companion in your kitchen, inspiring you to create culinary masterpieces that honor your Blood Type O identity. Here's to a future filled with vibrant health, culinary delights, and the endless possibilities that come with embracing the unique and beautiful you.

Bon appétit and continued well-being on your Blood Type O adventure!